AF207020

BECOME A
DIAGNOSTIC MEDICAL SONOGRAPHER

by Kari Cornell

BrightPoint Press

San Diego, CA

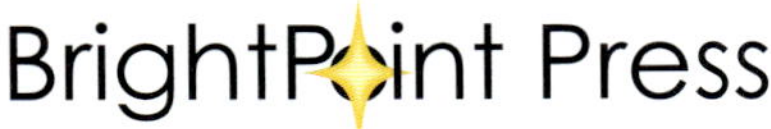

© 2025 BrightPoint Press
an imprint of ReferencePoint Press, Inc.
Printed in the United States

For more information, contact:
BrightPoint Press
PO Box 27779
San Diego, CA 92198
www.BrightPointPress.com

LIBRARY OF CONGRESS CATALOGING-IN-PUBLICATION DATA

Name: Cornell, Kari, author.
Title: Become a Diagnostic Medical Sonographer / by Kari Cornell.
Description: San Diego, CA: ReferencePoint Press, Inc., 2025 | Series: Skilled and Vocational Trades | Audience: Grade 10 to 12 | Includes bibliographical references and index.
Identifiers: ISBN: 9781678208967 (hardcover) | ISBN: 9781678208974 (eBook)
The complete Library of Congress record is available at www.loc.gov.

CONTENTS

AT A GLANCE

- Diagnostic medical sonographers use sound waves to take pictures of organs, muscles, and tissues. These are called ultrasound images or sonograms.

- Sonographers study the ultrasound images for signs of disease. They look for kidney stones, tumors, and other problems.

- Sonographers write reports about what they find on scans. These reports go in the patients' medical records.

- Sonographers must earn a 2-year or 4-year college degree. They also need to take a test to become a certified diagnostic medical sonographer.

- When they are students, sonographers do clinical work in hospitals, clinics, or labs. They learn how to take ultrasound scans and work with patients.

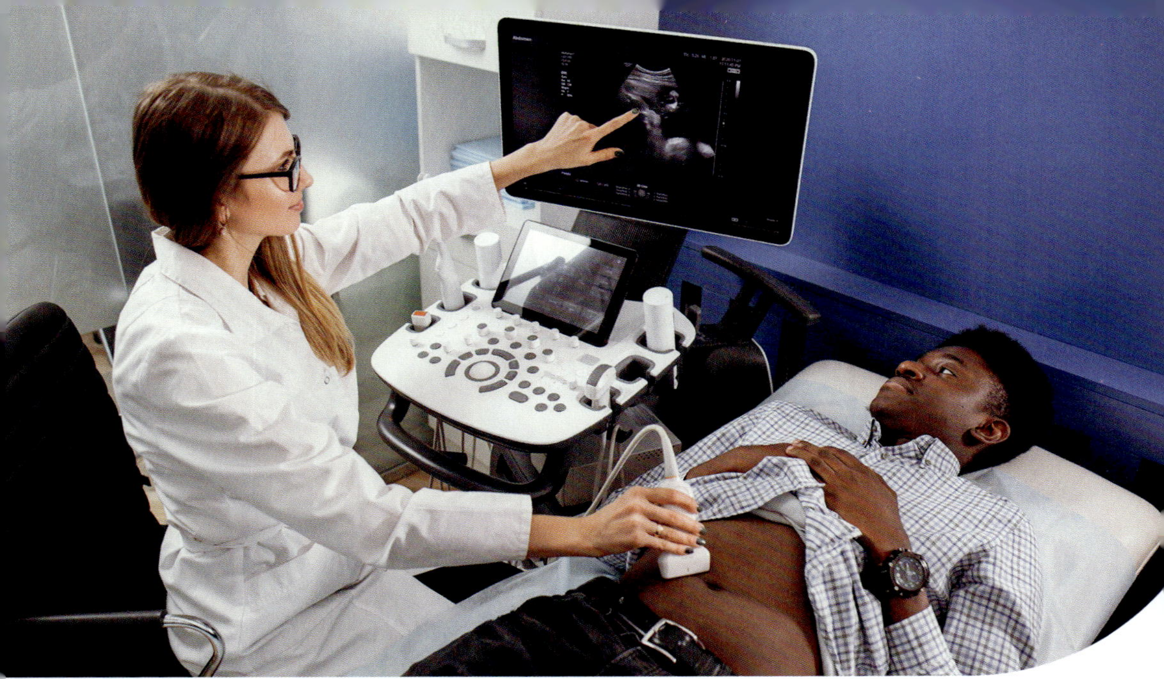

- Sonographers may specialize in different areas of the body. These areas might include the heart, blood vessels, female reproductive system, or muscles and bones.

- The field of diagnostic medical sonography is growing. Between 2022 and 2032, it is expected to grow by 14 percent.

- Ultrasound technology is advancing quickly. Small, handheld scanners are portable and easy to use.

HELPING TO SAVE LIVES

A woman was feeling unwell, and she went to the emergency room. The medical staff told her there was nothing wrong. They sent her home. But she still felt sick. She went to see her doctor. He also told her there was nothing to worry about. She still did not feel right. The woman made an appointment with Leigh Anne.

Leigh Anne is an echocardiographer. These medical professionals take pictures

It takes skill and practice to operate an ultrasound machine.

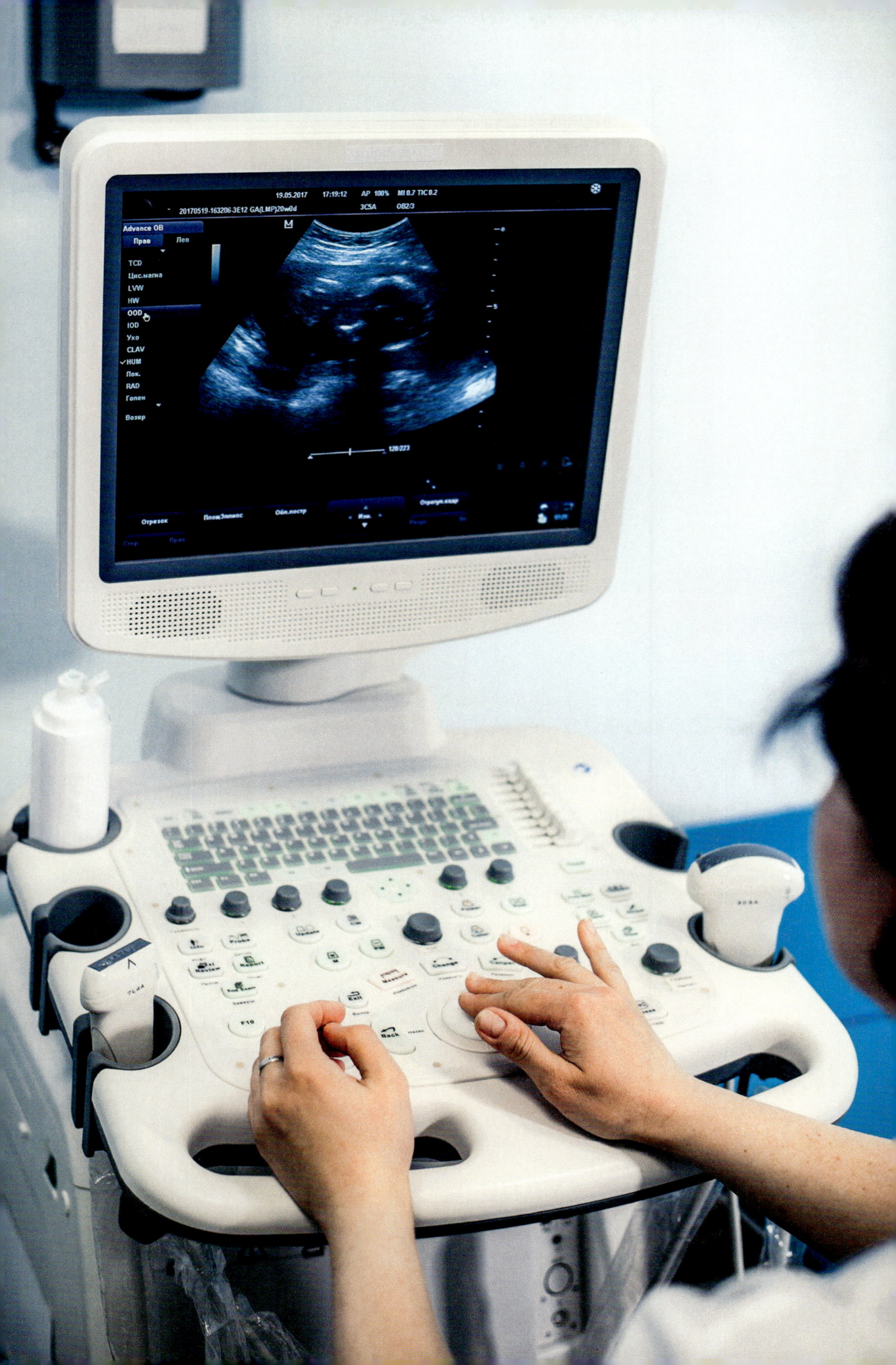

19.05.2017   17:19:12   AP 100%   MI 0.7 TIC 0.2
20170519-163206-3E12 GA(LMP)20w0d   3C5A   OB2/3
Advance OB
Прав   Лев
TCD
Цис.магна
LVW
HW
OOD
IOD
Ухо
CLAV
✓HUM
Лок.
RAD
Голен
Возвр
M
120/223
Отрезок   ПлощЭллипс   Обл.постр   Изм.   Открут.иззр
Стер   Прав

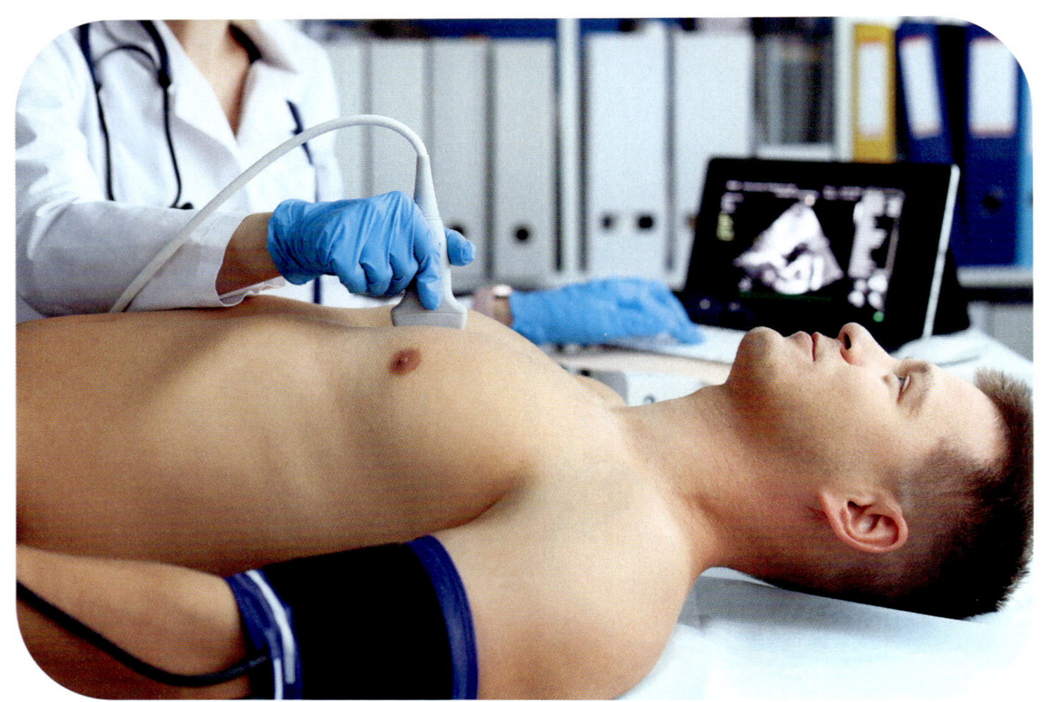

of the heart using sound waves. This process is called an ultrasound.

Leigh Anne took an ultrasound of the woman's heart. At first she thought it looked healthy. Then she noticed that the aorta looked too large. This is the main blood vessel that carries blood out of the heart. Leigh Anne took more pictures. She could see that the carotid artery had a tear in it.

This blood vessel carries blood up to the brain.

This was serious. If the woman had not seen Leigh Anne, she would have died within 2 days. The tear could have formed a **blood clot**. This clot could have stopped blood flow to the brain.

The patient was lucky. Leigh Anne found the problem just in time. The woman had surgery to repair the damaged vessel. Six months later, she visited Leigh Anne. "You saved my life," she said as she gave Leigh Anne a hug.[1]

WHAT IS A DIAGNOSTIC MEDICAL SONOGRAPHER?

The word *diagnostic* means identifying a disease. Sonographers use ultrasound

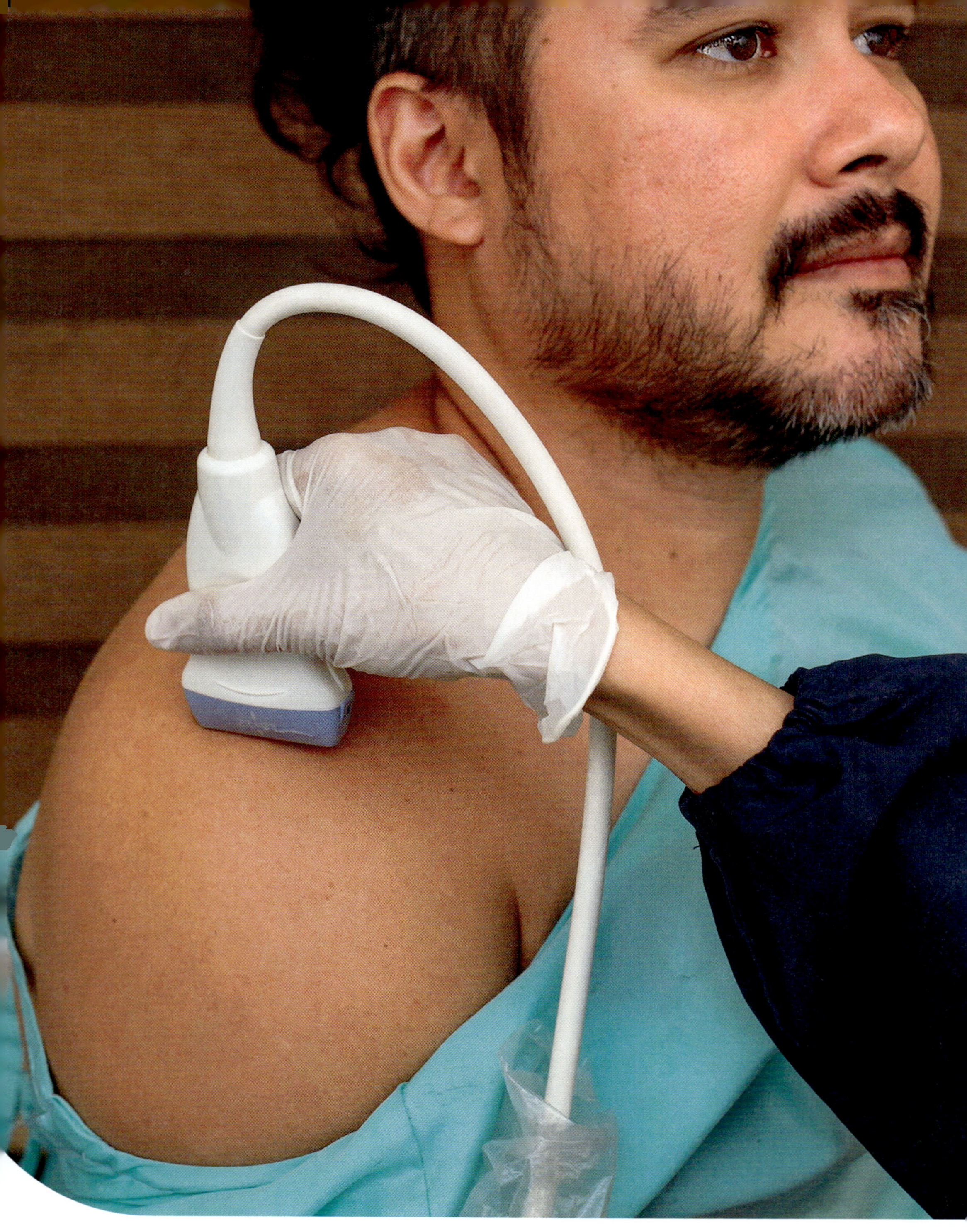

Ultrasounds can be used to check muscles
and tendons.

equipment to take images of the body. They use these images to learn why a patient is sick.

Diagnostic medical sonographers are often the first people to spot dangerous issues. Ultrasounds can reveal tumors, **abnormalities** in babies, and other problems. Doctors use this information to treat the patient. Sonographers play a key role in helping patients find answers.

CHAPTER ONE

WHAT DOES A DIAGNOSTIC MEDICAL SONOGRAPHER DO?

People often think of babies when they think of ultrasounds. Sonographers check the growth and development of unborn babies during pregnancy. But ultrasounds are also used in many other situations. They can be used to take images of blood flowing through the heart. Ultrasounds are often used to find gallstones. These are pebble-size pieces of material in the gallbladder that can

Ultrasounds are commonly performed on pregnant people, but they have many other uses too.

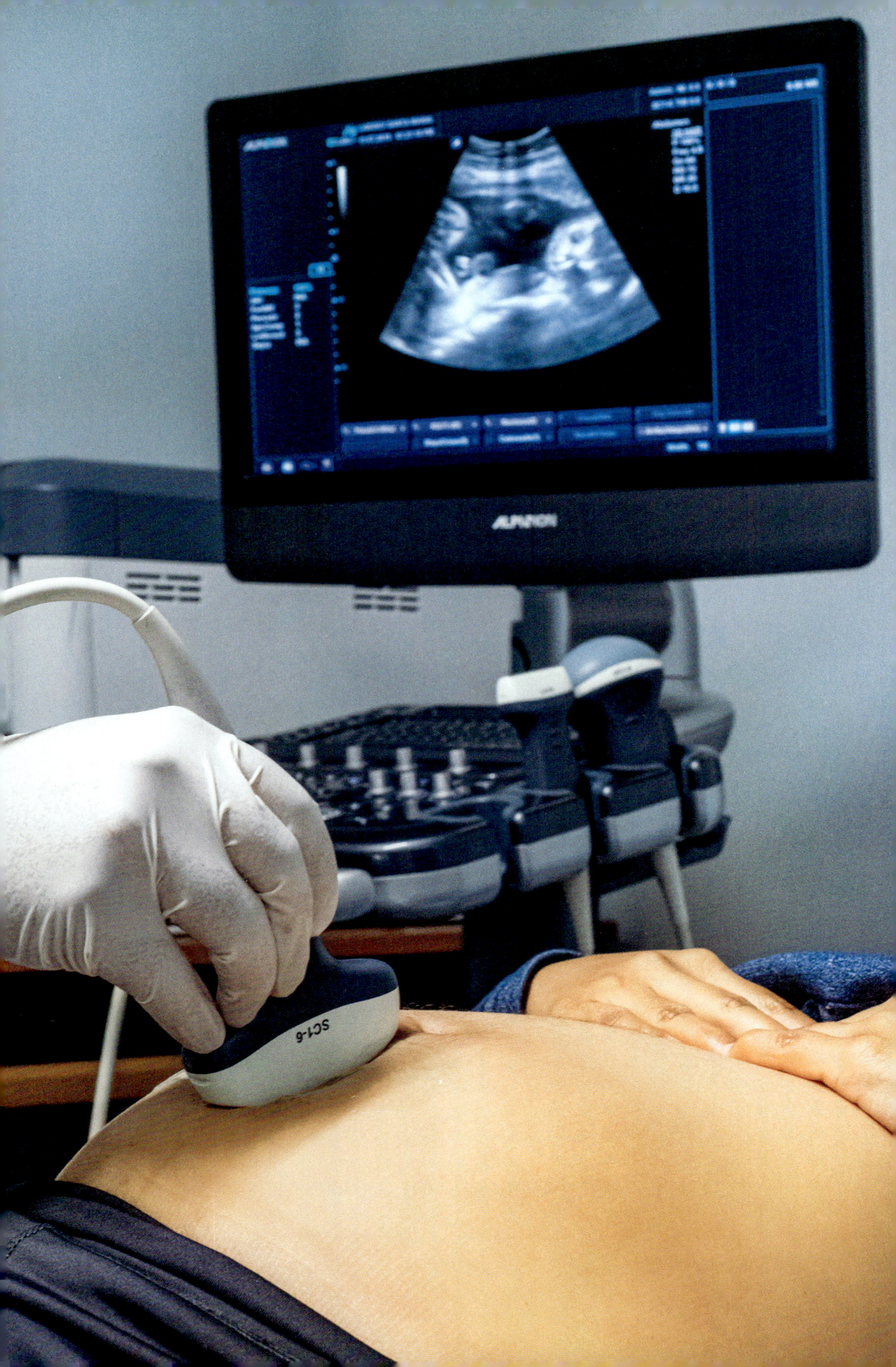

cause pain. They are formed from hardened bile, a liquid that helps digest food. Sonographers also use ultrasounds to study the eyes, chest, skin, and other parts of a patient's body.

HOW AN ULTRASOUND WORKS

To do an ultrasound, a sonographer holds a transducer against a patient. This is a wand with a flat end. The sonographer might apply a gel to the skin. This is done to stop air pockets from blocking the sound waves. The sonographer slowly runs the transducer along the skin. The device beams sound waves into the body. These sound waves are too high-pitched to hear.

The waves bounce off the tissues, muscles, and bones. They then reflect

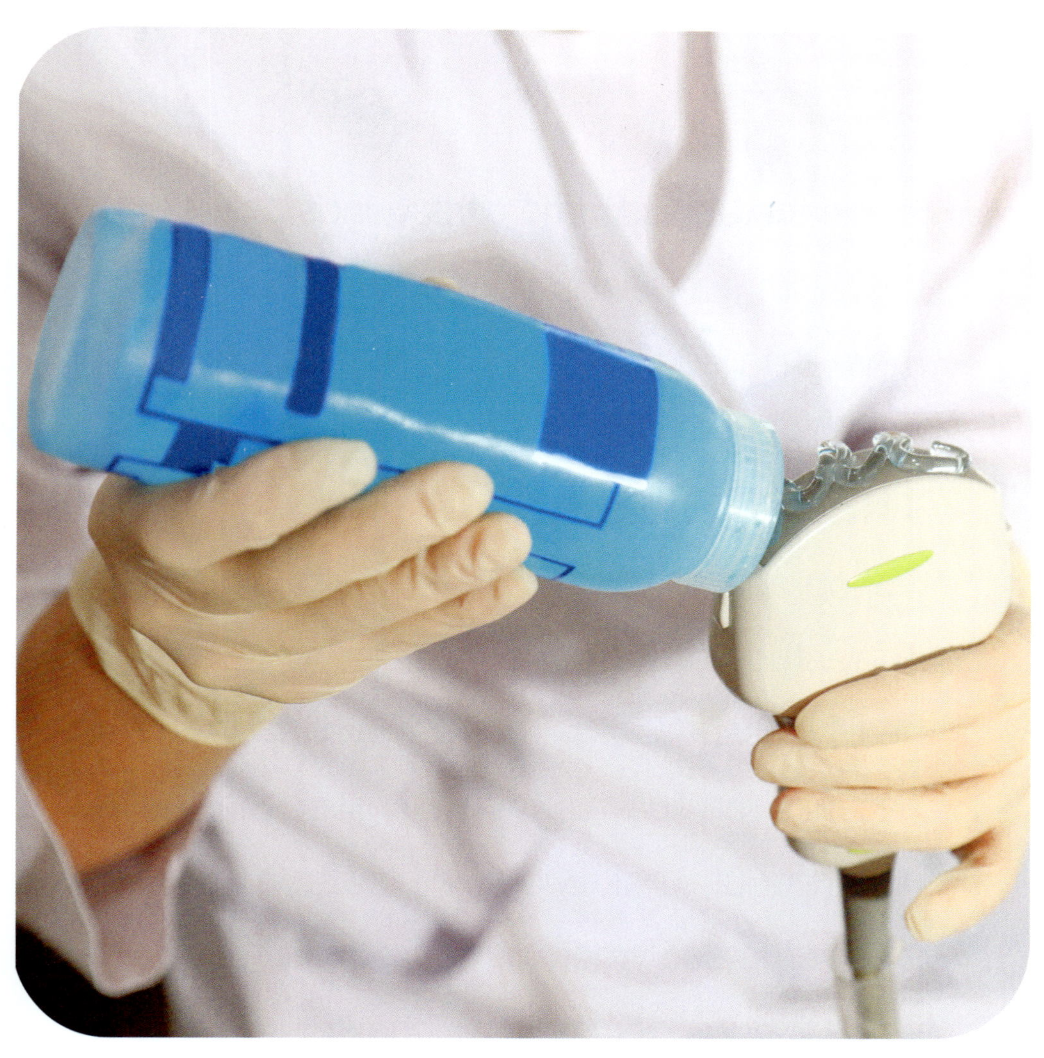

Using gel on the transducer results in better images.

back to the transducer. This produces
electrical signals that are sent to a
scanner. The scanner uses the timing of
the reflections to create a picture. The
picture shows the tissues and organs

inside the body. Some ultrasounds provide a two-dimensional image. Others show a more detailed three-dimensional picture.

THE FIRST TO KNOW

Sonographers look for anything unusual. They study **anatomy** so they know what healthy tissue looks like. They also learn the patient's medical history. This gives them clues about what to look for. It also makes it easier to see when something is wrong. The sonographer is usually the first to know about a health concern.

One sonographer described what this means to her. She said, "I have been the first person to see a **metastasis** in the liver. . . . What drives you to go to work each day is knowing that you're going to help someone get what they need to get healthy."[2]

Sonographers do not talk with the patient about what they see in the scans. That is the job of the doctor. The sonographer shares the images with the doctor.

Emotions

Keeping emotions in check is a challenge for sonographers. But it is important. Marlo Duffy explains, "We have to always remember that, although our day may be difficult, stressful, or busy, our patients are in the hospital. They are often very ill or going through what may be the most difficult times in their lives. Empathy and compassion go a long way when caring for patients."

"Explore 'A Day in the Life' of Two Diagnostic Medical Sonographers," Concorde, January 6, 2020. www.concorde.edu.

The doctor then uses the scans to develop a plan for how to care for the patient.

OTHER TASKS

Sonographers do more than take ultrasound images. They also prepare patients for the ultrasound. They explain

Keeping patients informed and comfortable is part of a sonographer's job.

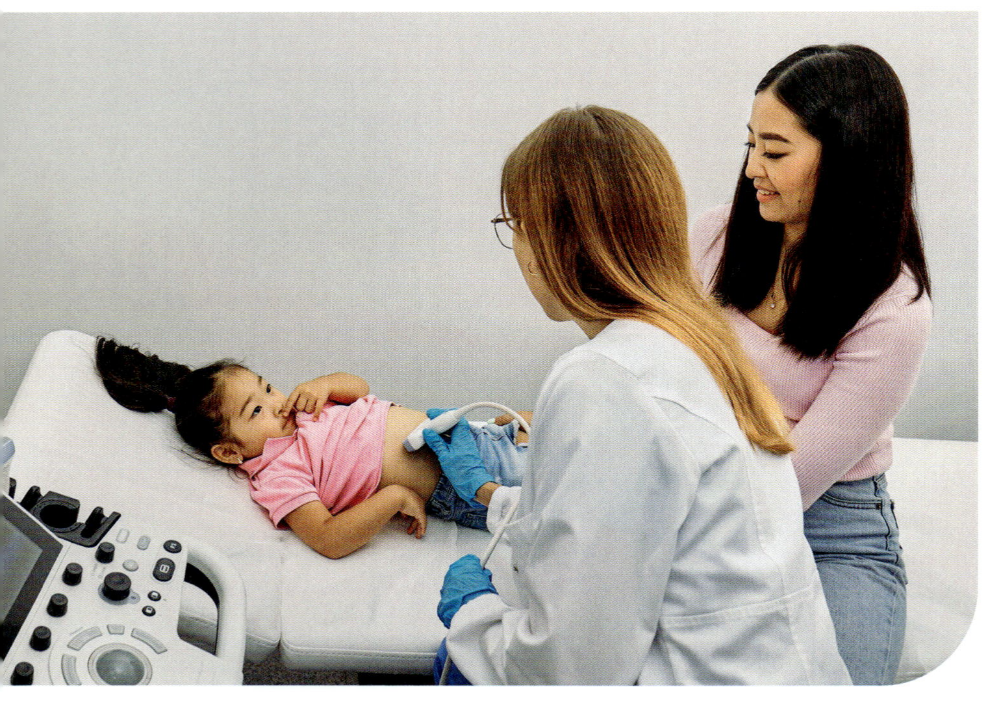

the process and answer questions.
Sonographers get the exam room ready.
They make sure the equipment is working
correctly. They keep records of scan results
and update patient files. Sonographers
work with doctors and with other
departments. They help arrange the next
steps for the patient's care.

Sonographers also help with biopsies.
A biopsy is a procedure in which tissue
is collected from a patient. The sample is
then studied in a lab to check for problems.
Anita Jennings describes this procedure.
She says, "We commonly assist physicians
with biopsies of the liver, breast, thyroid,
and many other organs. We guide the
physician's needle placement for fluid
drainage of the chest and abdomen. . . .

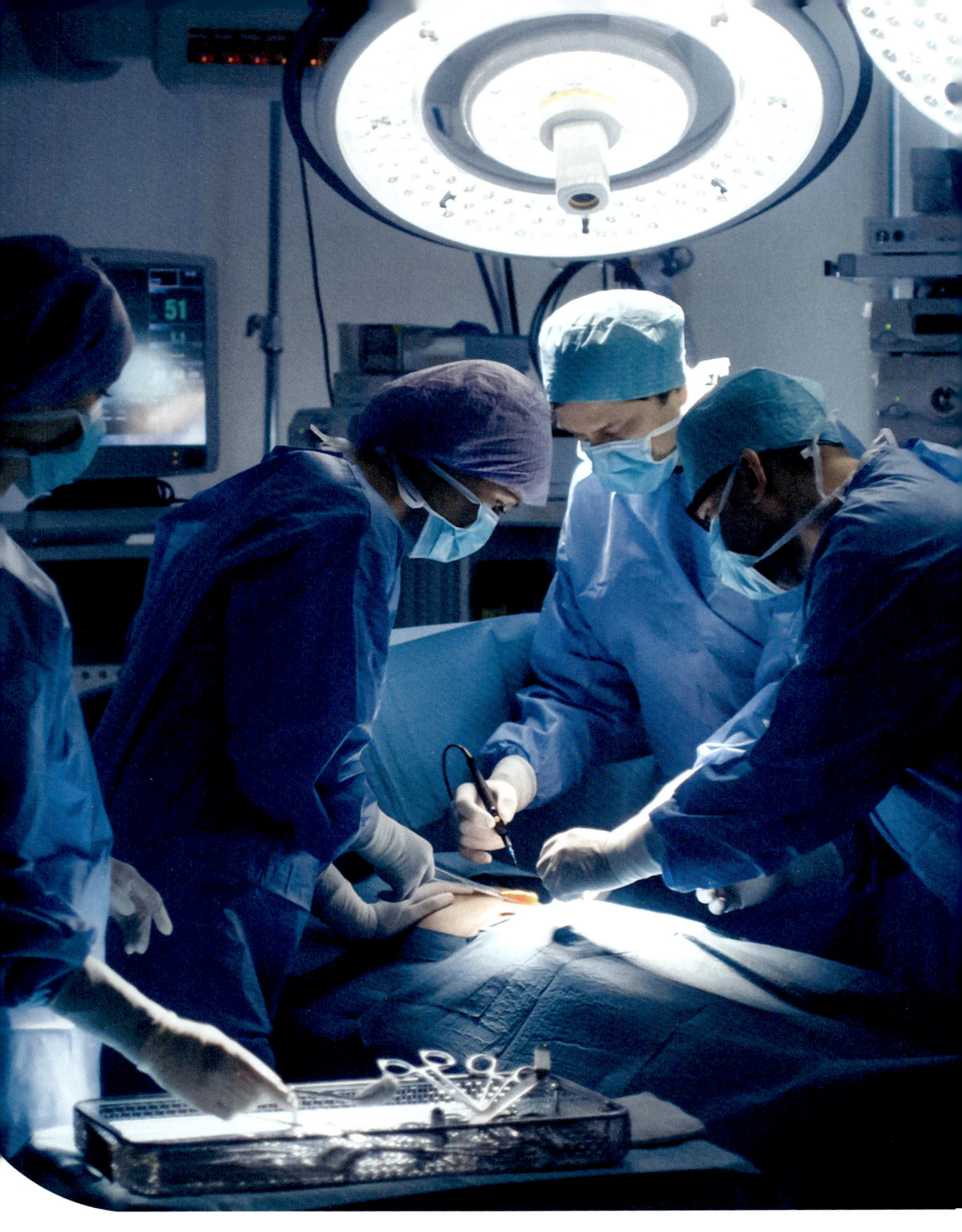

Sonographers are beginning to play a role in some operating rooms.

And when the procedures are done, we are responsible for dressing the wound and giving the patient their post-procedure care instructions."[3]

Sonographers also help in an operating room. They may scan the brain during surgery to find a tumor that needs to be removed. Or they may scan a liver in an opened abdomen. This helps surgeons avoid damaging blood vessels. This is a relatively new use for ultrasounds. "We are always learning, always growing," Jennings explains.[4]

CHAPTER TWO

WHAT TRAINING DO DIAGNOSTIC MEDICAL SONOGRAPHERS NEED?

A career in sonography usually begins with an interest in anatomy. Sonographers are also interested in medical care. They have technology skills. These workers need good hand-eye coordination to operate ultrasound machines. They tend to be curious and precise. They pay careful attention to details. This helps them notice problems on a scan.

Good knowledge of anatomy is key for sonographers.

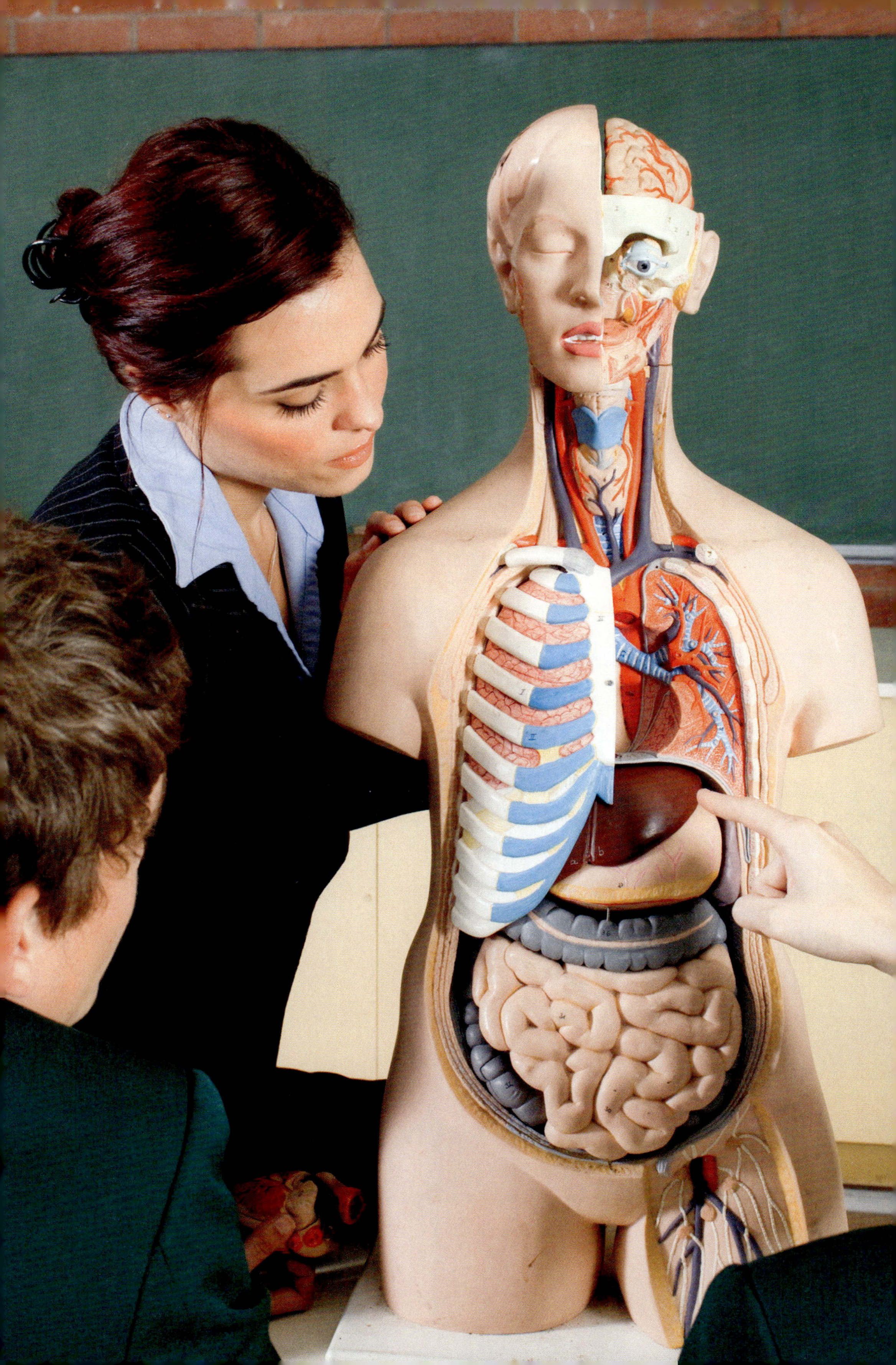

Most important, sonographers like working with patients. They want to help patients get better. They are driven to get patients the care they need. One sonographer described what it takes to do the job. They said, "A successful sonographer is someone who has an independent personality, who is bright, has strength of character and a strong

Get a Jump Start

Students can take classes in high school that will prepare them for sonography. Anatomy, biology, physiology, chemistry, math, and physics are all helpful. If a student enjoys these classes, sonography may be a good career fit for them. Studying these subjects in high school can also give students an advantage when they enter college.

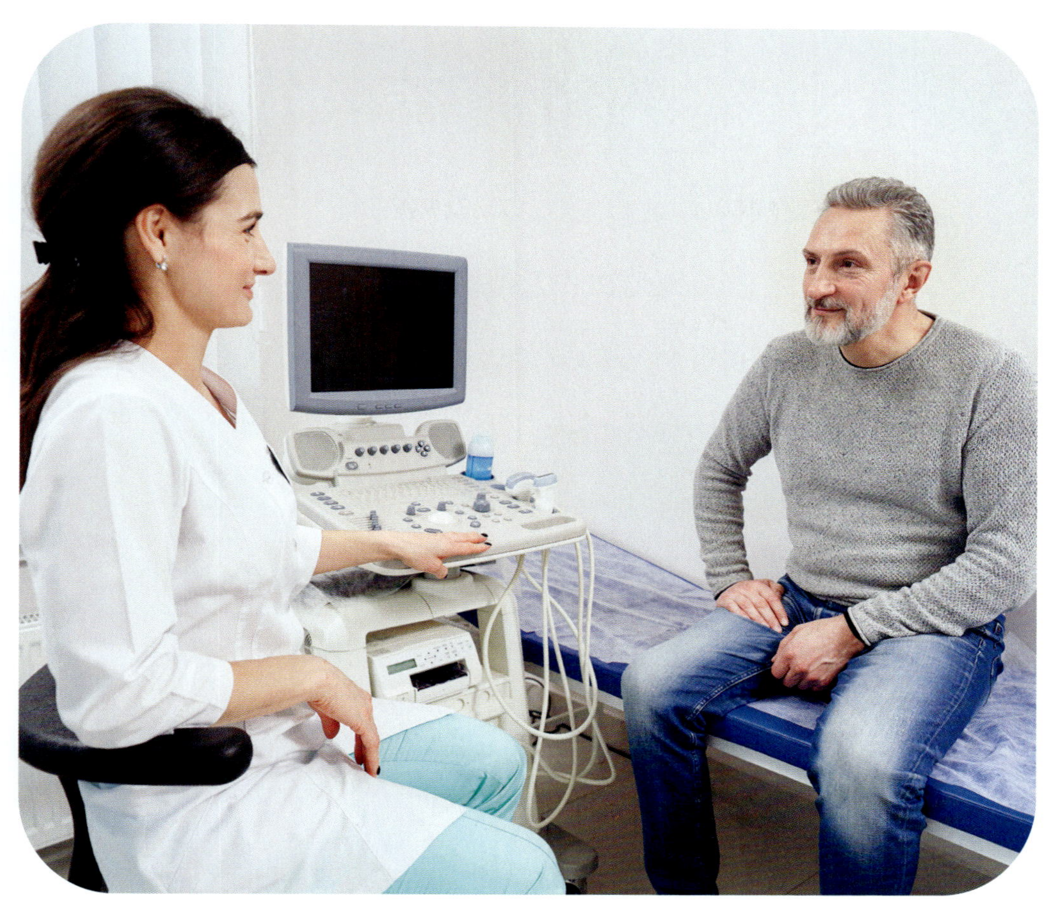

Sonographers meet many new people on a daily basis.

ethical background. It is also important
to . . . enjoy working with and dealing
with people."[5]

EARNING A DEGREE

Diagnostic medical sonographers must
have a college degree. Two-year and 4-year

colleges offer degrees in sonography. Sonography students start by studying anatomy and physiology. Anatomy covers the body's structures. Physiology covers how those structures work. Students also study biology, physics, chemistry, and math. There are many new words to learn. Those who work in hospitals or clinics must take a class in medical **terminology**.

As part of their studies, students do clinical work. This means they work full time for 12 months. Clinical work takes place at hospitals, clinics, and laboratories. Students learn how to use ultrasound equipment. They spend many hours working with professional sonographers. The sonographers show the students exactly

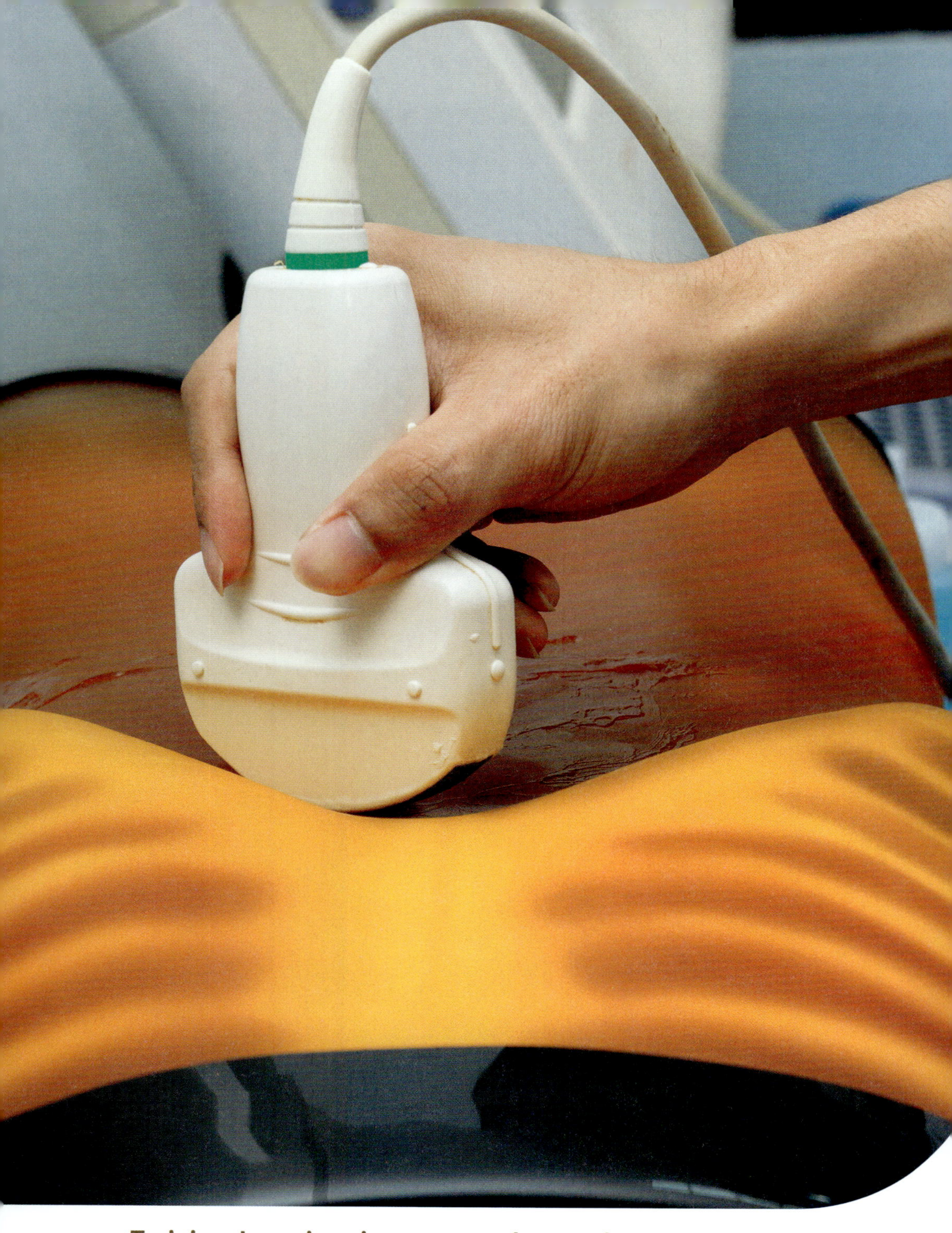

Training dummies give sonographers a chance to practice their skills before seeing real patients.

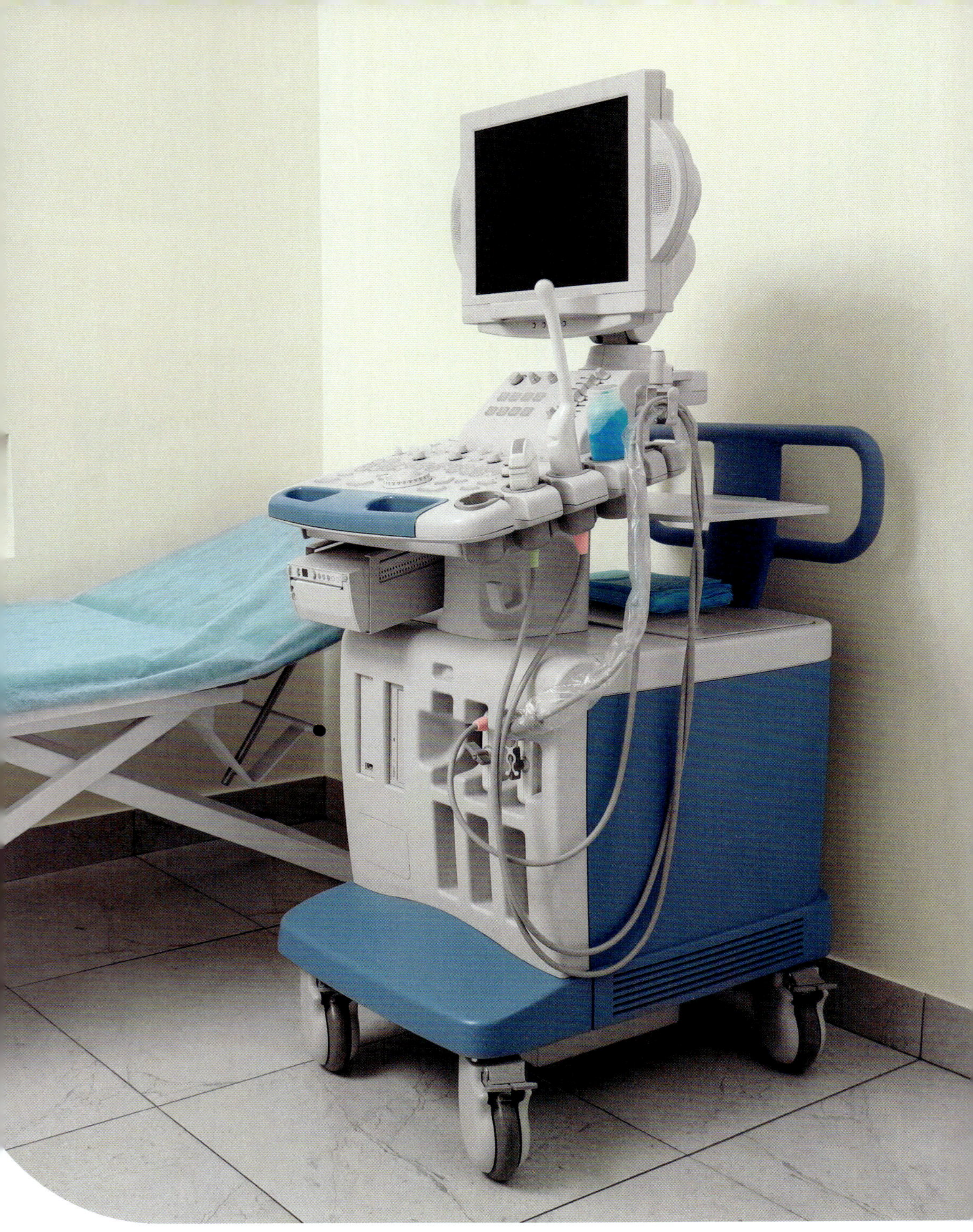

Ultrasound machines are complex devices that may cost tens of thousands of dollars.

what to look for on the scans. The students also learn how to interact with patients.

SPECIALIZING

When students have finished their general classes, they focus on a **specialization**. Colleges offer different sonography specializations. Some students may work with the heart. They will learn how to take an echocardiogram. This is a video of the heart as it is pumping. It is used to study the size of the heart. Sonographers see if the blood is flowing properly. They check whether the heart valves are working as they should.

There are many other specialties. **Musculoskeletal** sonography looks at muscles and bones. Neurosonography

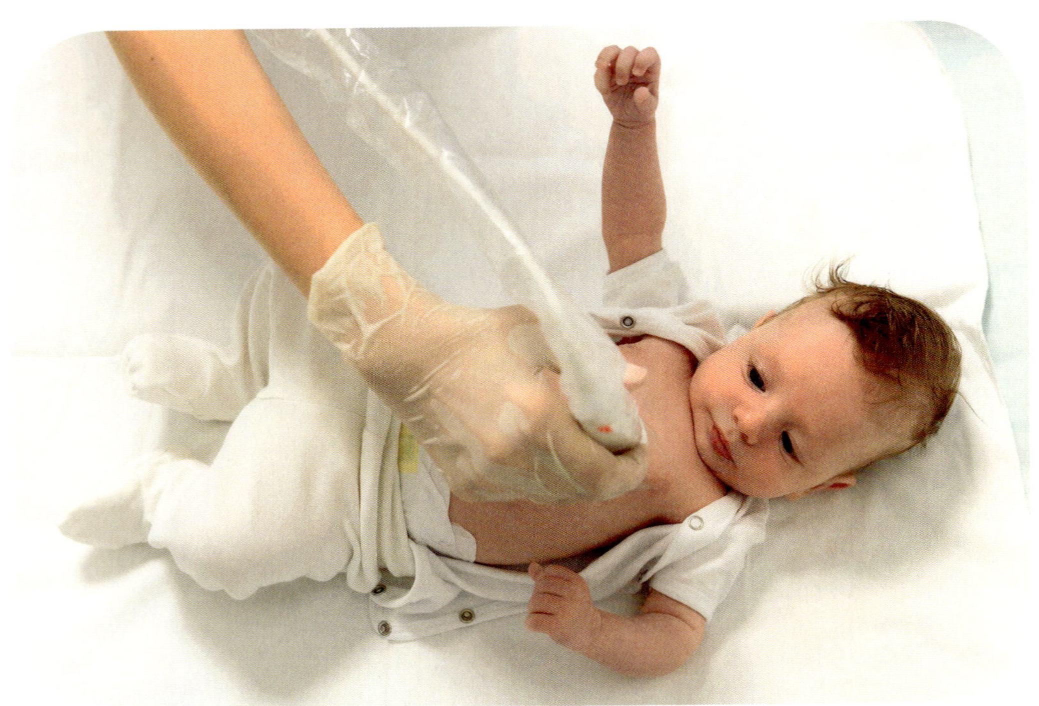

Some sonographers specialize in ultrasounds on very young patients.

studies the brain and nervous system.
Abdominal sonography focuses on the
abdomen. Gynecologic sonography
looks at a woman's reproductive system.
Breast sonographers scan breast tissue.
Pediatric sonographers specialize in doing
ultrasounds on children.

Specializing provides a chance to learn
something new. One person in the field

explained, "This is a career that tests your expertise daily and changes from moment to moment. . . . It also affords you the opportunity to grow within the field, by acquiring certification in multiple specialties, so that you can broaden or focus your expertise, as desired."[6]

CERTIFICATION

After completing a college degree, students enter a 1-year certification program. Many colleges, universities, and teaching hospitals offer these programs. Certification involves more classes. Students learn more about how to operate the equipment. They get more experience in reading the results. They also practice caring for patients in a clinical setting.

Sonographers are required to take basic life support training as well. This training includes cardiopulmonary resuscitation (CPR). CPR is done when a person's heart has stopped beating. Chest compressions are used to try to restart the heart. Mouth-to-mouth breathing may be done to push air into the person's lungs.

At the end of the program, students must take a test. The test has two parts. The first is about ultrasound tools and concepts. The second is about an ultrasound specialty. Students can choose from many different options. Some people specialize in the abdomen or breast. Fetal echocardiography is another option. This means taking scans of an unborn baby's heart.

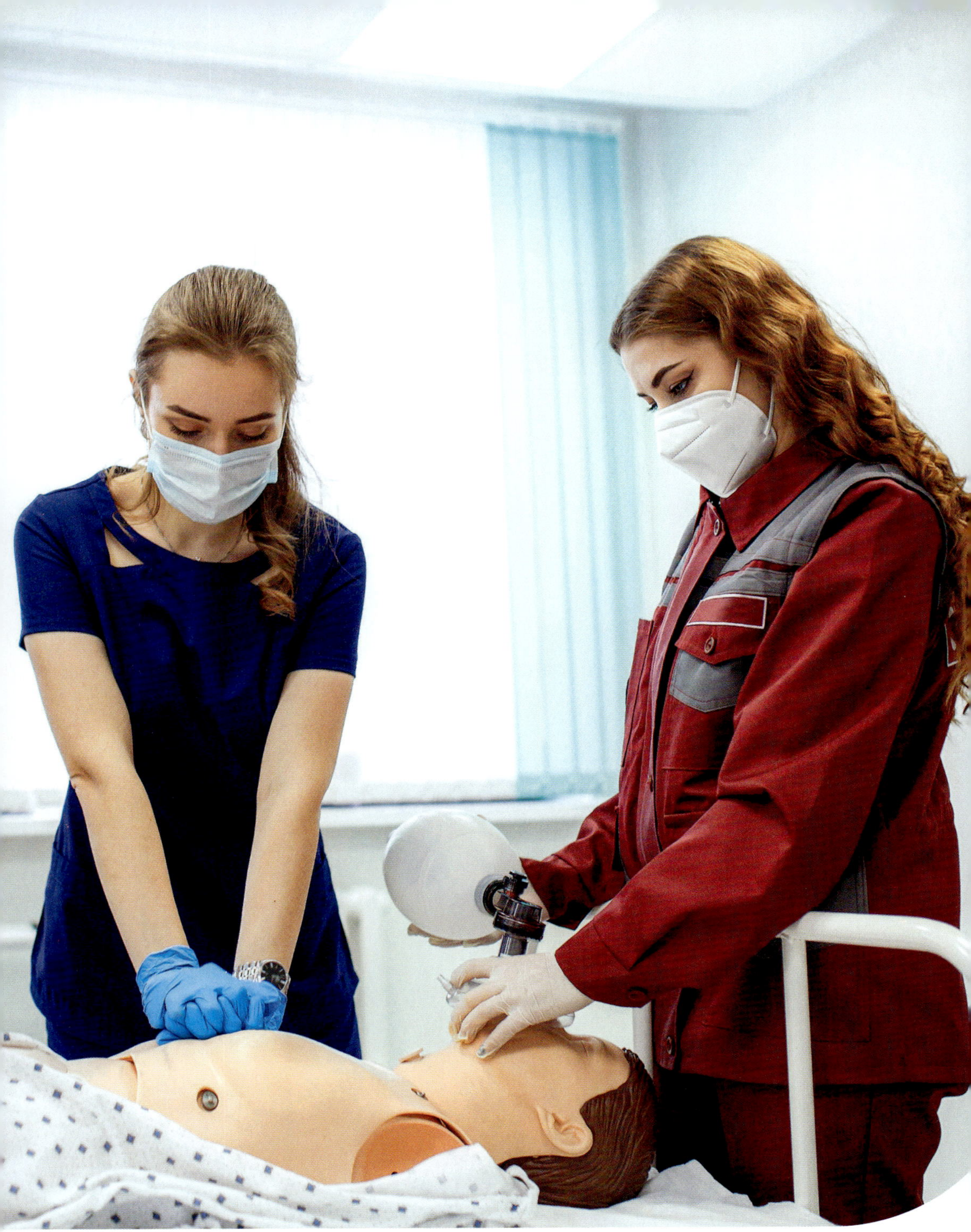

CPR training is important for many medical professionals, including sonographers.

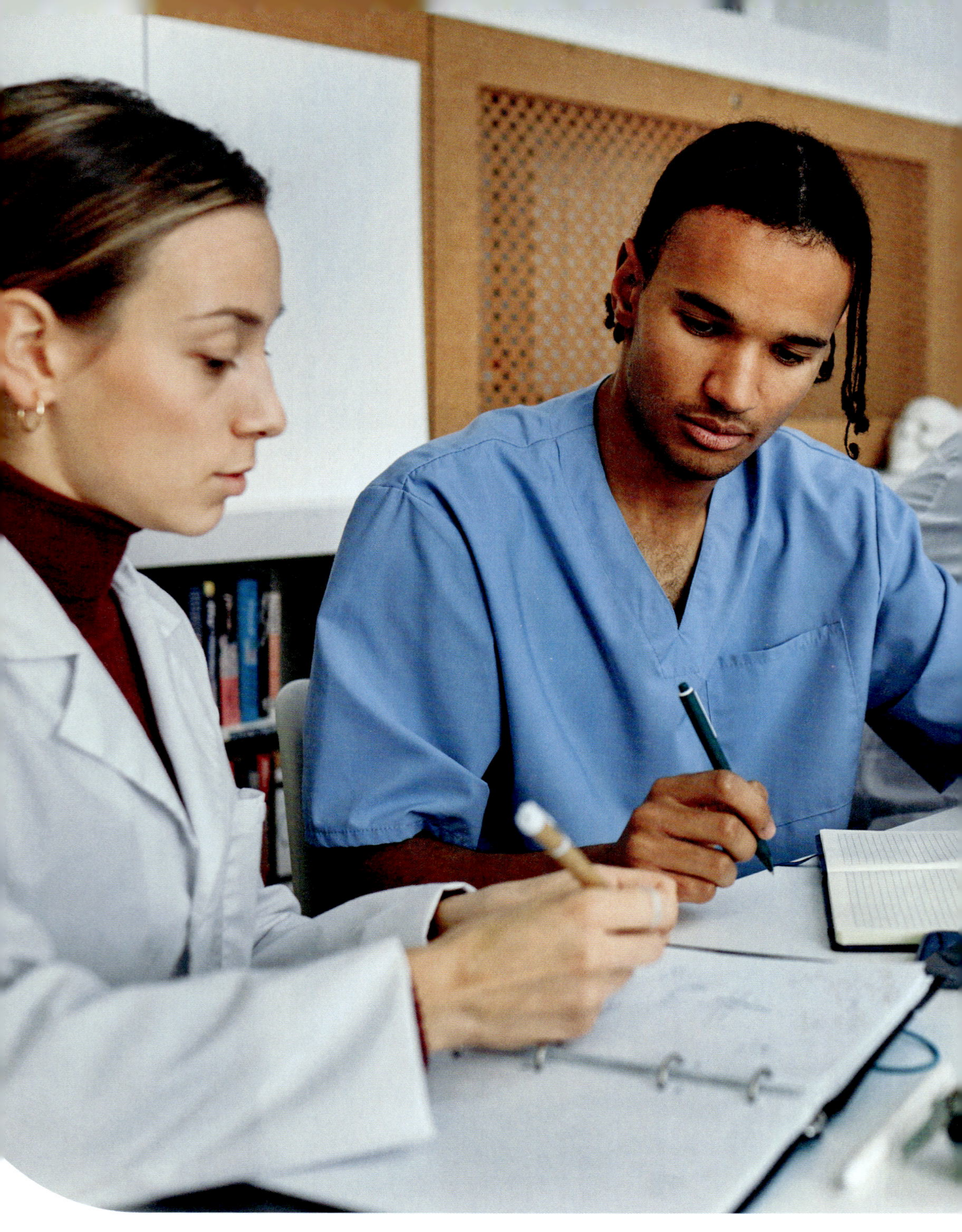

Continuing education helps sonographers refresh their skills and learn about new advances.

These tests are run by the American Registry for Diagnostic Medical Sonography (ARDMS). By passing the tests, students become certified. Becoming certified is not required, but it may help sonographers get a job. There are additional tests for further specialization. Many sonographers become certified in more than one specialty.

Sonographers must continue to take classes to stay certified. They must take at least thirty credits every 3 years. Each class is between three and five credits. These classes are called continuing medical education (CME) requirements. They help sonographers keep their knowledge up to date.

CHAPTER THREE

WHAT IS LIFE LIKE AS A DIAGNOSTIC MEDICAL SONOGRAPHER?

Many diagnostic medical sonographers say their work is rewarding. One explained, "I enjoy what I do because I get the chance to talk to diverse people. I get to help them, and share in their positive and negative experiences. . . . Some feel that the good results are the most rewarding, such as sharing a moment with an expectant mom; however, when I find a large complication and can then help the

Helping patients is a rewarding part of being a sonographer.

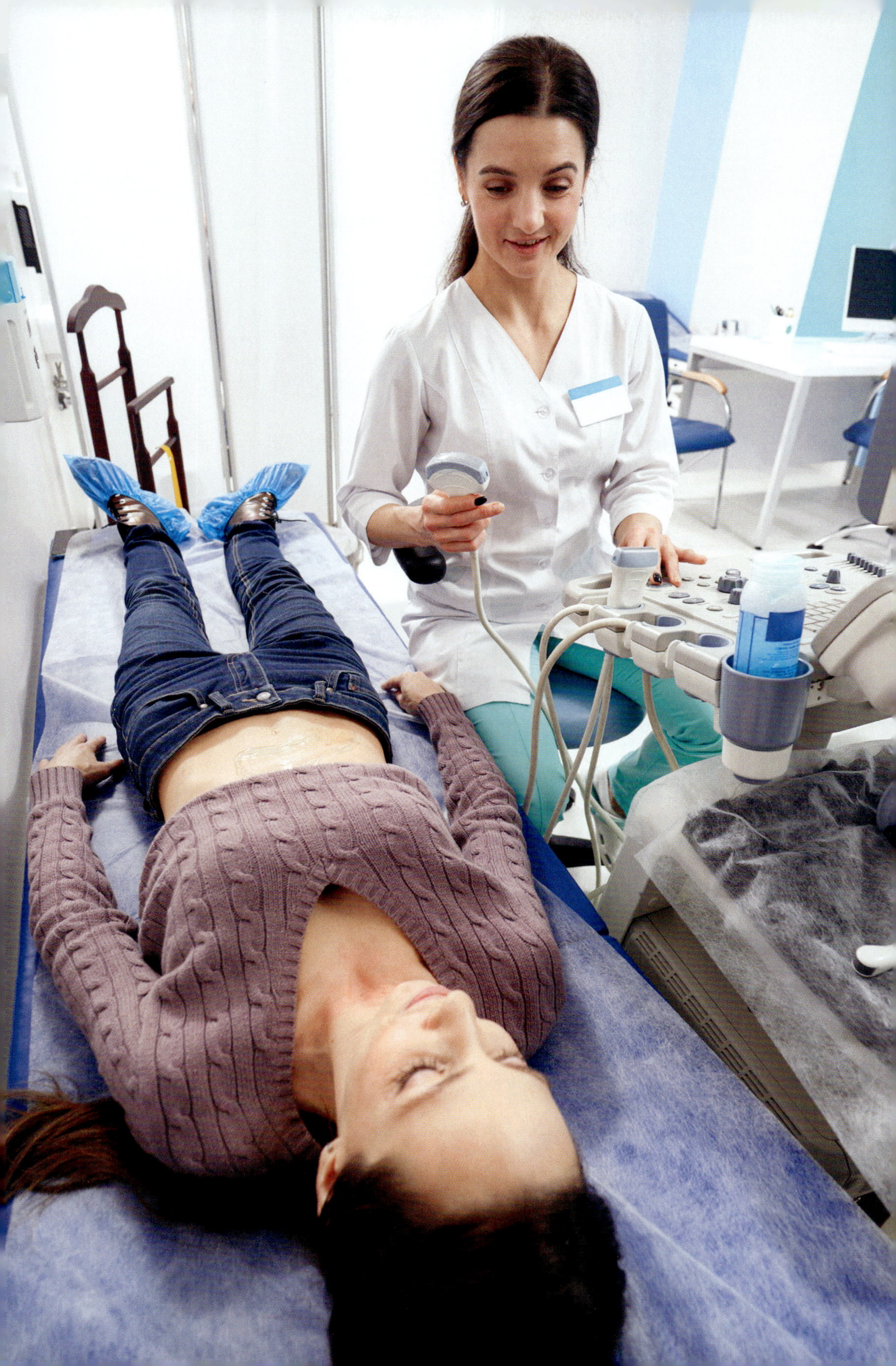

patient and be there for them . . . that is the
most rewarding for me."[7]

Sonographers may work in a clinic,
hospital, emergency room, or lab. Most
work full time. They spend up to 12 hours
a day on their feet. Sonographers in a
hospital usually work in a room just for
ultrasounds. Those in an emergency room
take scans at a patient's bedside. Basic
ultrasound equipment may be a handheld

Being on Call

Sometimes sonographers are on call. They can
stay home, but they have to be ready to go in
to work. If called in, they need to arrive at work
within 30 minutes. In other cases, a sonographer
may leave work only to be called back later to do
an emergency ultrasound.

scanner connected to a laptop. Bigger units may be on a cart. Sonographers wheel them from one patient to the next.

STARTING THE DAY

The typical day for medical sonographers is busy. As soon as they get to work, they check the schedule. They learn what scans they will be doing. Sonographers may perform more than fifteen ultrasounds in one shift. Sometimes more scans are added during the day. This might mean working overtime.

Sonographers pull up the chart for each patient. They look to see what kind of scan has been ordered. Sonographers read what kind of symptoms the patient has had. For instance, a sonographer might see that they are scheduled to do a gallbladder scan. The patient has been having abdominal pain.

Sonographers take the patient's weight and check **vital signs**. They also take the patient's blood pressure. Blood pressure is the amount of force caused by blood pushing against the walls of the arteries.

Sonographers may use a tablet to check medical records as they talk to patients.

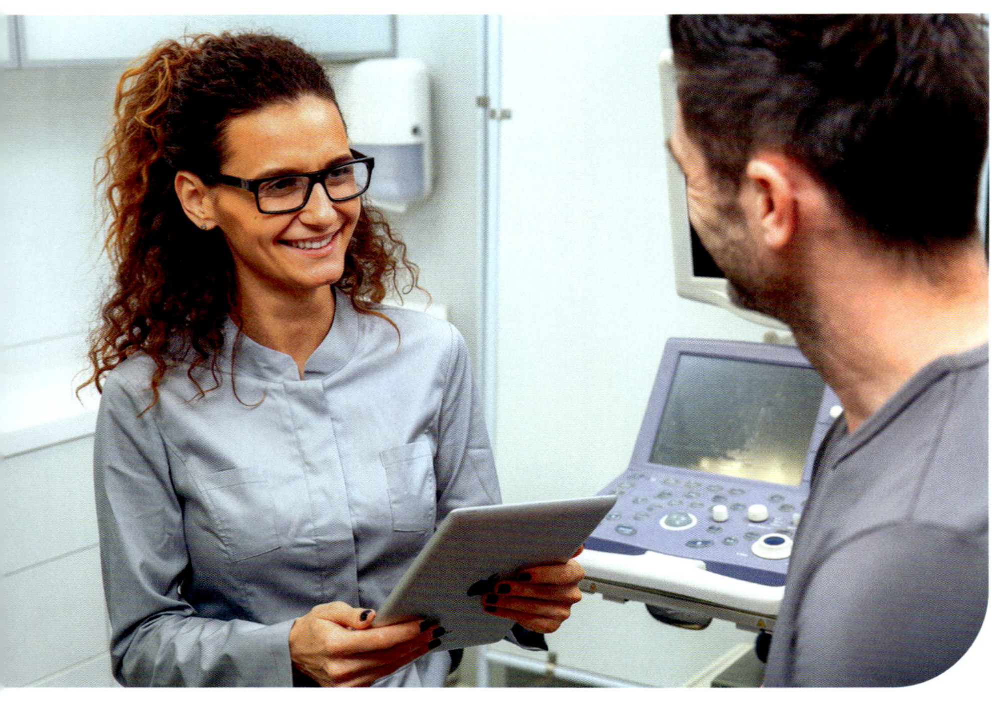

Sonographers then talk with the patient. They discuss the patient's medical history. They ask about new symptoms. Then they give the patient a hospital gown. They describe how they will do the scan.

COMPLETING THE SCAN

When the patient is ready, the sonographer returns to do the scan. For a gallbladder test, the sonographer will scan the liver, pancreas, bile duct, right kidney, and gallbladder. They make sure the patient is comfortable. Then they apply a warm gel to the skin. They guide the transducer along the patient's abdomen. As they scan, they watch the screen carefully. They are checking the organs for anything that

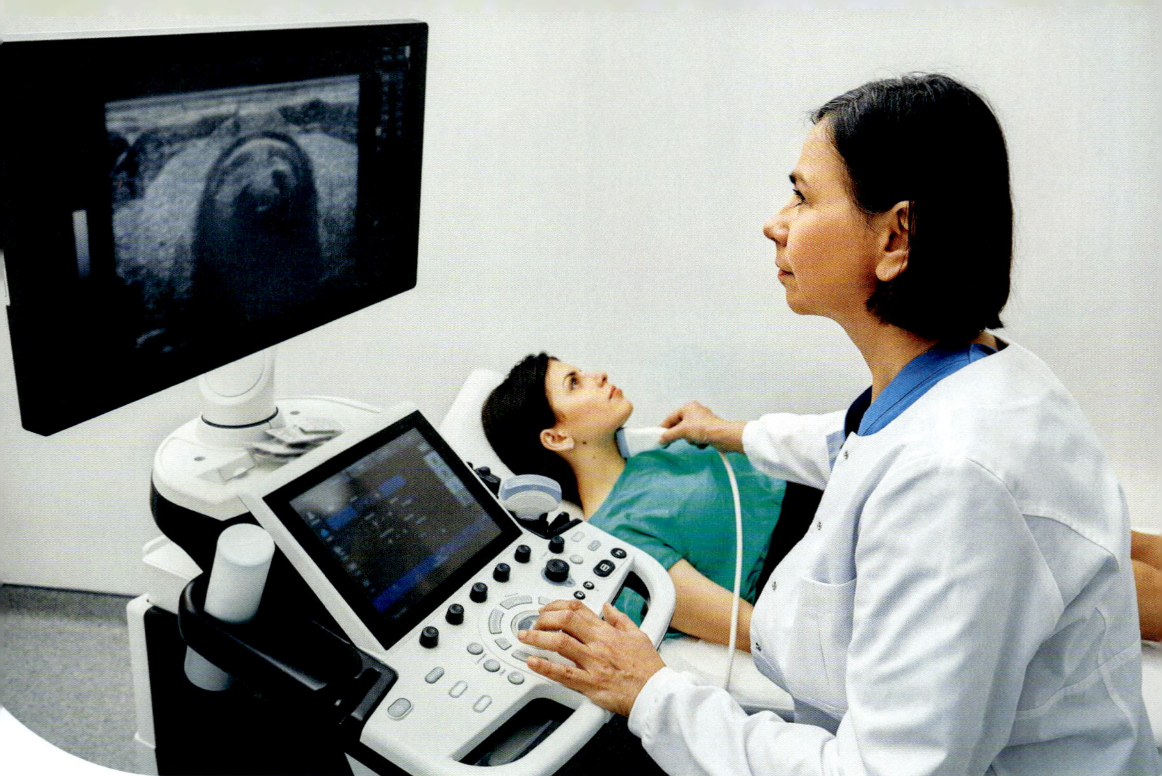

Sonographers are trained to interpret what they see on the ultrasound screen.

looks unusual. They check the texture of the pancreas. They look for gallstones.

Once the scan is complete, sonographers ask if the patient has any questions. They explain the next steps. Then sonographers fill out a report. They include details about any unusual findings. If the scan is clear, the sonographer will add "WNL" to the chart. This means "within normal limits." The sonographer discusses the results of the scan with the doctor. The first scan of the day is done. There may be many more to come.

RISKS AND POTENTIAL DANGERS

Being a medical sonographer is not easy. Going through the same motions all day can lead to repetitive strain. These are injuries from doing the same motion over and over. Other types of scans, such as X-rays, can expose workers to harmful radiation. But operating an ultrasound machine is safe. The sound waves are not dangerous to the sonographer or the patient.

Working as a sonographer can be tiring. Sonographers have a fast-paced schedule. They spend many hours on their feet.

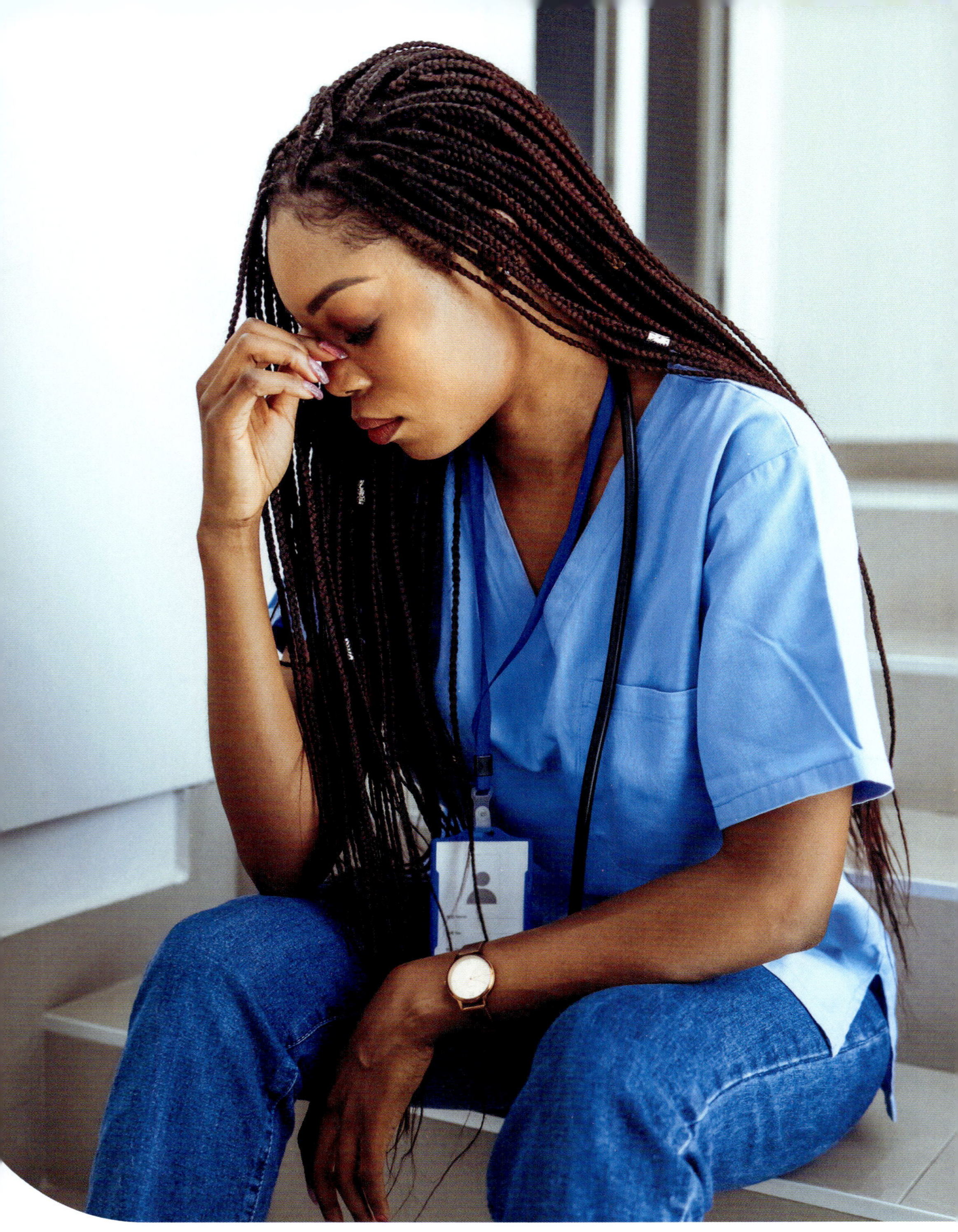

As with many medical jobs, being a sonographer can be physically and emotionally challenging.

Overtime may be needed if more scans are added throughout the day. A sonographer's job can be emotionally tiring as well. A big part of the job is seeing the results of the ultrasound. Bad news can cause emotional stress.

CHAPTER FOUR

WHAT IS THE FUTURE FOR DIAGNOSTIC MEDICAL SONOGRAPHERS?

The future for diagnostic medical sonographers is bright. The US population is aging. This means more sonographers will be needed. They can help **diagnose** issues common in older adults, such as heart disease. Additionally, more patients are looking for imaging options that are safer than X-rays.

The US Bureau of Labor Statistics (BLS) is a government agency. It collects

The sonography field is expected to continue growing in the future.

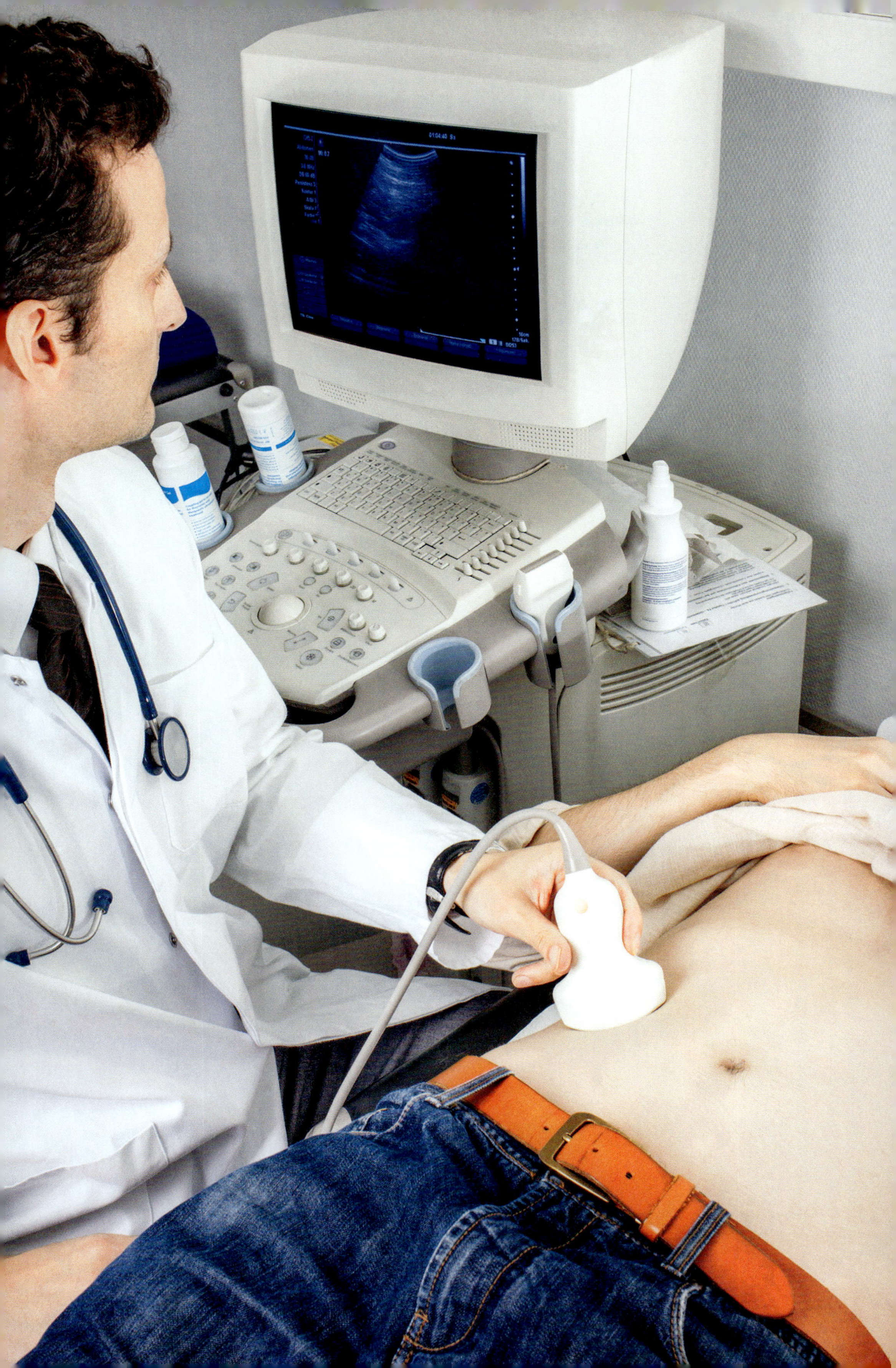

SONOGRAPHERS BY STATE

State	Employment	Employment per thousand jobs	Annual mean wage
California	8,100	0.46	$114,480
Texas	6,590	0.51	$78,440
Florida	6,470	0.70	$74,110
New York	5,910	0.65	$89,340
Ohio	3,650	0.68	$77,250

Source: "Occupational Employment and Wage Statistics," Bureau of Labor Statistics, 2022, *https://bls.gov.*

The five states with the most sonographer jobs are California, Texas, Florida, New York, and Ohio.

information about many careers. It found that there were 83,800 diagnostic medical sonographers in the United States in 2022. The agency also makes predictions about career growth in the future. The BLS estimates the need for sonographers will grow by 14 percent between 2022 and 2032.

The BLS provides information about salaries, too. Its data shows that diagnostic medical sonography pays well. In 2022, the average salary for this job was $81,350. For all other occupations, the average pay that year was $46,310.

TECHNOLOGICAL ADVANCES

As the need for ultrasounds increases, the technology is improving. Small handheld units are replacing large older machines. They are even replacing laptop units. Artificial intelligence (AI) has made it possible to capture quality ultrasound images using smartphones or tablets. These systems are precise and easy to use. They provide reliable results. AI can also reduce the number of false positives. A false positive is when people think a scan shows a disease, but it really doesn't.

Advances like these mean ultrasounds will be available to more patients. Experts predict that handheld units will help doctors diagnose heart disease during annual checkups. Learning to use these devices may become part of basic medical training. Ultrasounds may even be done at home. They could be used to monitor atrial fibrillation. This is an irregular heartbeat. At-home ultrasounds may also help with treating fertility issues and monitoring diseases.

And experts predict ultrasound devices will get even smaller. Scanners may be no bigger than a watch. This portability could be life-changing. Professor Joseph Osterwalder says, "The future lies in personalised ultrasound. This means a

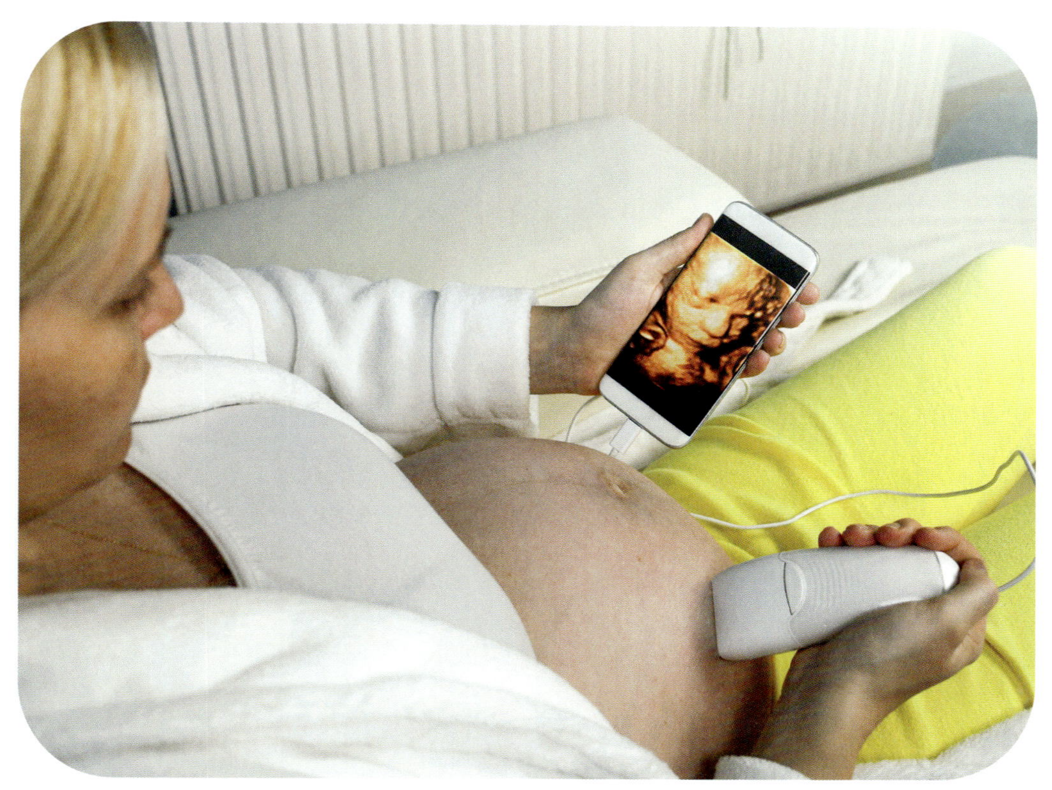

Portable devices that work with smartphones are changing the world of ultrasound scanning.

doctor carries his/her own ultrasound scanner in their coat pocket. Ultrasound will take over from the stethoscope."[8]

Engineers at the Massachusetts Institute of Technology (MIT) are already making the personal ultrasound a reality. They've invented ultrasound stickers that can be attached to the body. The stickers are the size of a postage stamp. They record images of organs for 48 hours. Those wearing the stickers can run, jump, and move. The stickers stay in place. This allows doctors to watch the organs during activity.

In a test, people wearing the patches lifted weights. Doctors could see bright patterns in the muscles. This was damage caused by stress. In the future, the patches could be used to alert users when to stop exercising to avoid soreness.

MIT engineering professor Xuanhe Zhao explains what's next. He says, "We envision a few patches adhered to different locations on the body, and the patches would communicate with your cellphone, where AI algorithms would analyze the images on demand."[9] The goal is to get the stickers to work wirelessly. The team hopes that one day stickers like these will be for sale at local pharmacies. The stickers would be designed to monitor specific health conditions.

SUPPORTIVE COMMUNITY

The sonographer community is supportive. Those drawn to this field are passionate

Beyond Diagnostics

Ultrasound can be used for more than taking images. It can also be used to treat disease. Sound waves can be targeted to dissolve kidney stones. A similar technique can be used to break down tumors on the liver. And low-intensity ultrasound may speed up the healing of broken bones.

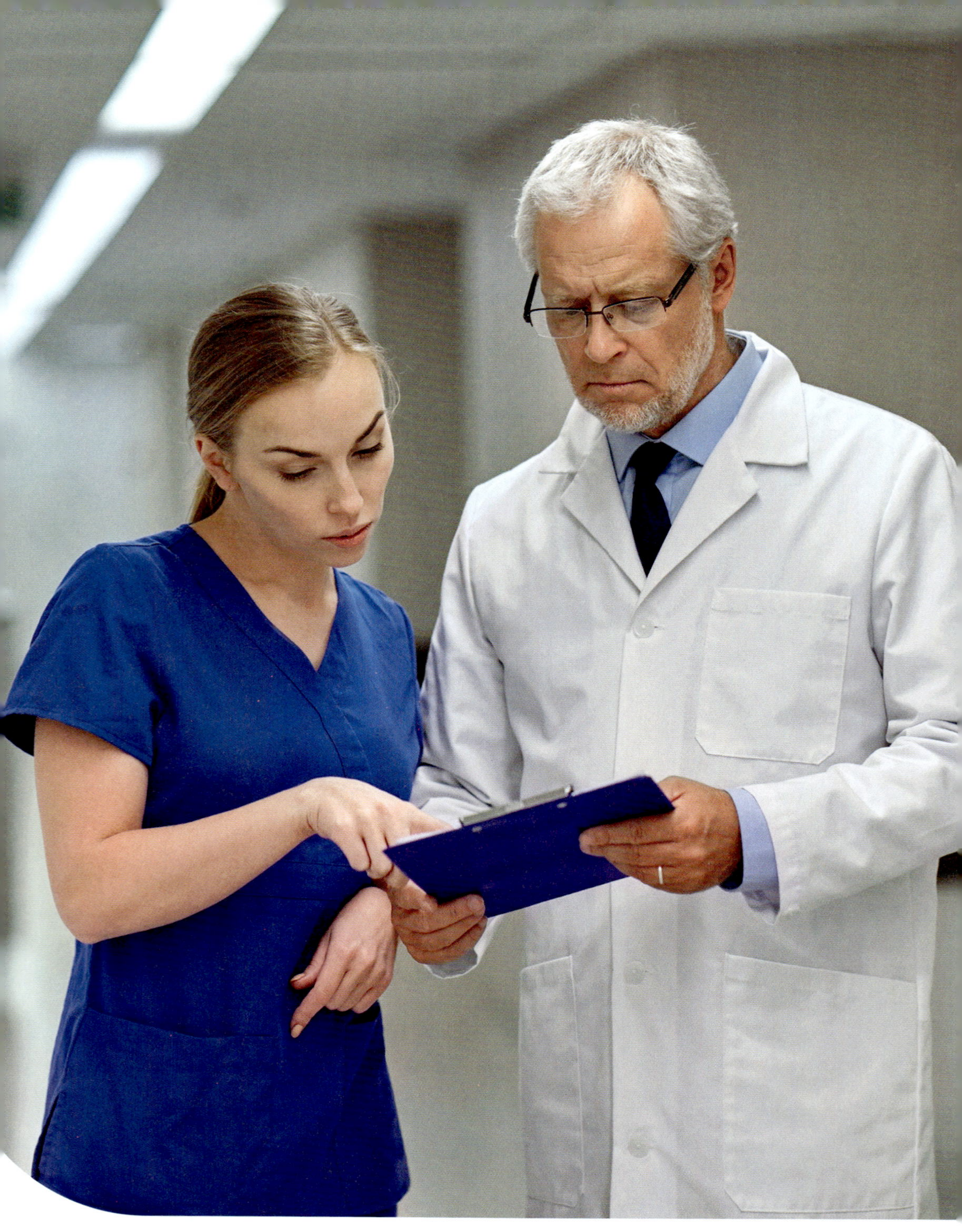

Mentors help to shape the next generation of sonographers.

about what they do. They want to share that passion with others. They also want to help grow the profession. Many sonographers help train the next generation by teaching classes. Others act as mentors. They pass along information to new sonographers. Longtime sonographer Sharlette was asked what she was most proud of in her career. She responded that it was the students she had mentored.

Advancing technology and the aging population will make diagnostic medical sonography a promising career path for years to come. The field may be a good fit for those who are interested in medicine, driven to help others, and able to embrace new tools. The future of the field will be shaped by tomorrow's sonographers.

As one sonographer observed, "The field of ultrasound is relatively young . . . as someone working in the field, you can play a role in where the profession goes."[10]

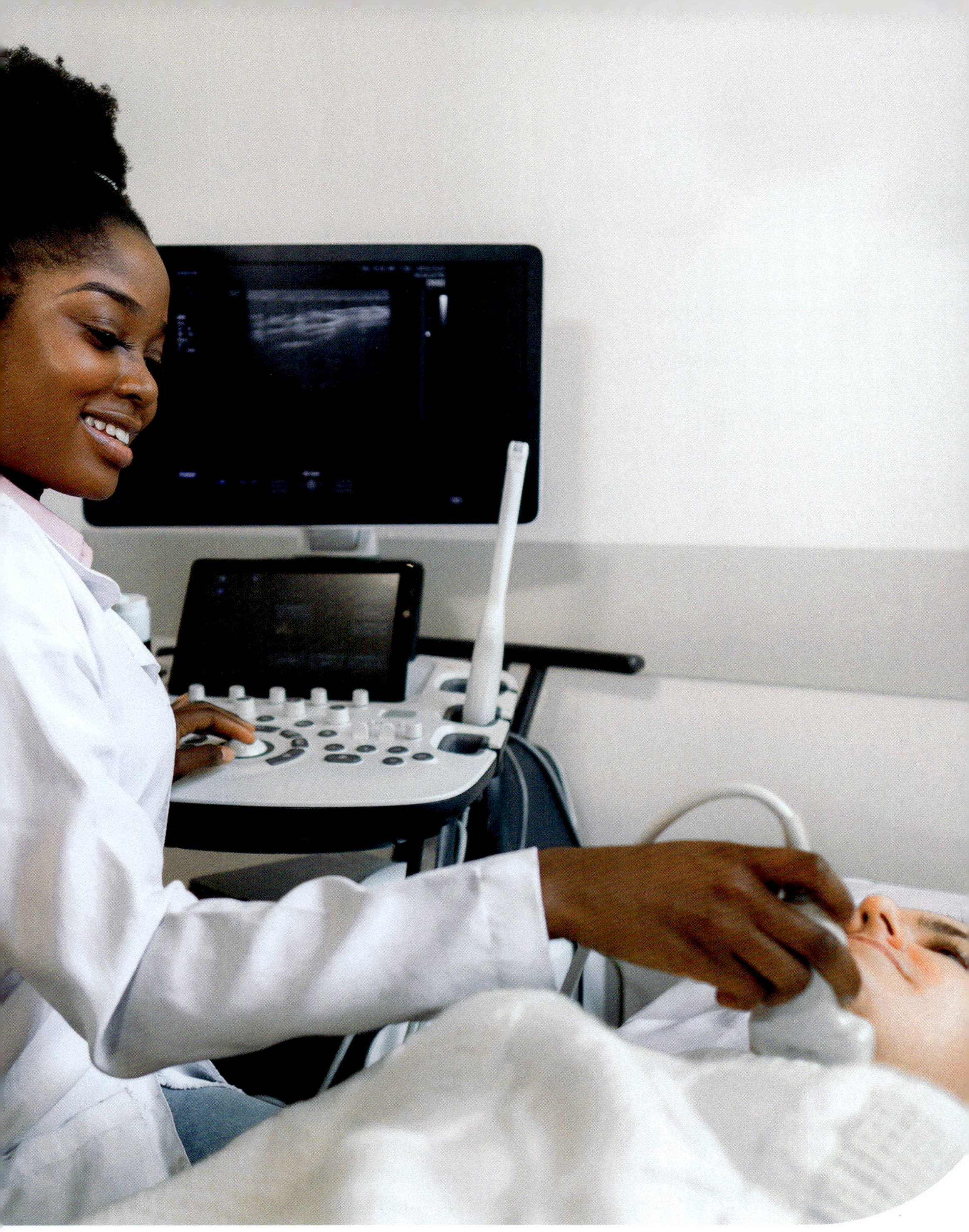

Sonographers get the chance to have a positive impact on their patients' lives.

GLOSSARY

abnormalities
things that are not normal

anatomy
the study of the parts of the human body

blood clot
a thick clump of blood that blocks blood flow through vessels

diagnose
to use signs and symptoms to identify a disease

metastasis
the spread of a disease from one part of the body to another

musculoskeletal
relating to the muscles and skeleton

specialization
to focus on a particular area in a field of work or study

terminology
a set of special words used in a particular field

vital signs
measurements of the body's basic functions, including temperature, heart rate, and breathing rate

INTRODUCTION: HELPING TO SAVE LIVES

1. Quoted in "Episode #3 of RealTalkSonography: Is There a Patient You'll Never Forget?" *YouTube*, uploaded by ARDMS, April 2, 2019. www.youtube.com.

CHAPTER ONE: WHAT DOES A DIAGNOSTIC MEDICAL SONOGRAPHER DO?

2. Quoted in "Episode #2 of RealTalkSonography: If Your Career Were to End, What Would You Be Most Proud of?" *YouTube*, uploaded by ARDMS, March 5, 2019. www.youtube.com.

3. Quoted in "Explore 'A Day in the Life' of Two Diagnostic Medical Sonographers," *Concorde*, January 6, 2020. www.concorde.edu.

4. Quoted in "Explore 'A Day in the Life' of Two Diagnostic Medical Sonographers."

CHAPTER TWO: WHAT TRAINING DO DIAGNOSTIC MEDICAL SONOGRAPHERS NEED?

5. Quoted in "Sonographer Testimonials," *ARDMS*. www.ardms.org.

6. Quoted in "Sonographer Testimonials."

CHAPTER THREE: WHAT IS LIFE LIKE AS A DIAGNOSTIC MEDICAL SONOGRAPHER?

7. Quoted in "Sonographer Testimonials."

CHAPTER FOUR: WHAT IS THE FUTURE FOR DIAGNOSTIC MEDICAL SONOGRAPHERS?

8. Quoted in "Explore 'A Day in the Life' of Two Diagnostic Medical Sonographers."

9. Quoted in Jennifer Maki, "The Future of Ultrasound and You!," *Anderson College*, September 29, 2021. www.andersoncollege.com.

10. Quoted in "Sonographer Testimonials."

FOR FURTHER RESEARCH

BOOKS

Emma Huddleston, *Work in the Health Care Industry*. San Diego, CA: BrightPoint Press, 2020.

Tamika M. Murray, *Become a Dental Hygienist*. San Diego, CA: BrightPoint Press, 2023.

Alice Roberts, *The Complete Human Body: The Definitive Visual Guide*. New York: DK, 2023.

INTERNET SOURCES

Ohad Arazi, "These 5 Predictions Will Shape the Future of Ultrasound Technology and Patient Care," *Fast Company*, January 9, 2023. www.fastcompany.com.

Jennifer Chu, "MIT Engineers Develop Stickers That Can See Inside the Body," *MIT News*, July 28, 2022. www.news.mit.edu.

B.J. Kim, "A New Vision for Ultrasound Imaging," *MIT News*, July 24, 2023. www.news.mit.edu.

WEBSITES

American Registry for Diagnostic Medical Sonography (ARDMS)
www.ardms.org

The ARDMS tests and certifies sonographers. Its website provides information about educational opportunities and jobs. It also includes testimonials from and interviews with practicing sonographers.

Cleveland Clinic: Ultrasound
www.my.clevelandclinic.org/health/diagnostics/4995-ultrasound

The Cleveland Clinic's website provides an in-depth overview of what an ultrasound is, how it's performed, and what information the tests can provide.

Society of Diagnostic Medical Sonography (SDMS)
www.sdms.org

This is the largest professional organization for sonographers in the world. SDMS's mission is to support, educate, and provide a network for sonography educators, students, and professionals.

INDEX

IMAGE CREDITS

Cover: © Africa Studio/Shutterstock Images
5: © Desizned/Shutterstock Images
7: © Roman Kosolapov/Shutterstock Images
8: © H_Ko/Shutterstock Images
10: © MDV Edwards/Shutterstock Images
13: © Uriel Perez/Shutterstock Images
15: © New Africa/Shutterstock Images
18: © Peakstock/Shutterstock Images
20: © Gorodenkoff/Shutterstock Images
23: © michaeljung/Shutterstock Images
25: © Yakobchuk Viacheslav/Shutterstock Images
27: © Kittipong Somklang/Shutterstock Images
28: © New Africa/Shutterstock Images
30: © Andrey Zhernovoy/Shutterstock Images
33: © Arlou_Andrei/Shutterstock Images
34: © SeventyFour/Shutterstock Images
37: © Yakobchuk Viacheslav/Shutterstock Images
40: © Lebedev Roman Olegovich/Shutterstock Images
42: © Peakstock/Shutterstock Images
44: © Dragana Gordic/Shutterstock Images
47: © mapman/Shutterstock Images
48: © Red Line Editorial
51: © TPROduction/iStockphoto
54: © Ground Picture/Shutterstock Images
57: © SofikoS/Shutterstock Images

ABOUT THE AUTHOR

Kari Cornell is an award-winning children's book author who gardens, runs, and makes pottery. She lives in Minneapolis with her husband, two boys, and their sweet dog, EmmyLou.